Printed in the United States of America
Sunny Day Publishing, LLC
ISBN 978-0-9825480-5-9

The Chubby Grasshopper

and His Two Friends

A story by Shelly Krajny

Illustrations by Melissa Cimino

Dedication

*To my parents, Charles and Deborah Jack,
and
Grandparents, John and Josephine Ferko,
for your continuous love and support.*

Shel Smith: You make my heart smile. Loya.

*Special thanks to all the remarkable
people in my life, who inspire greatness
in me and everyone around them.*

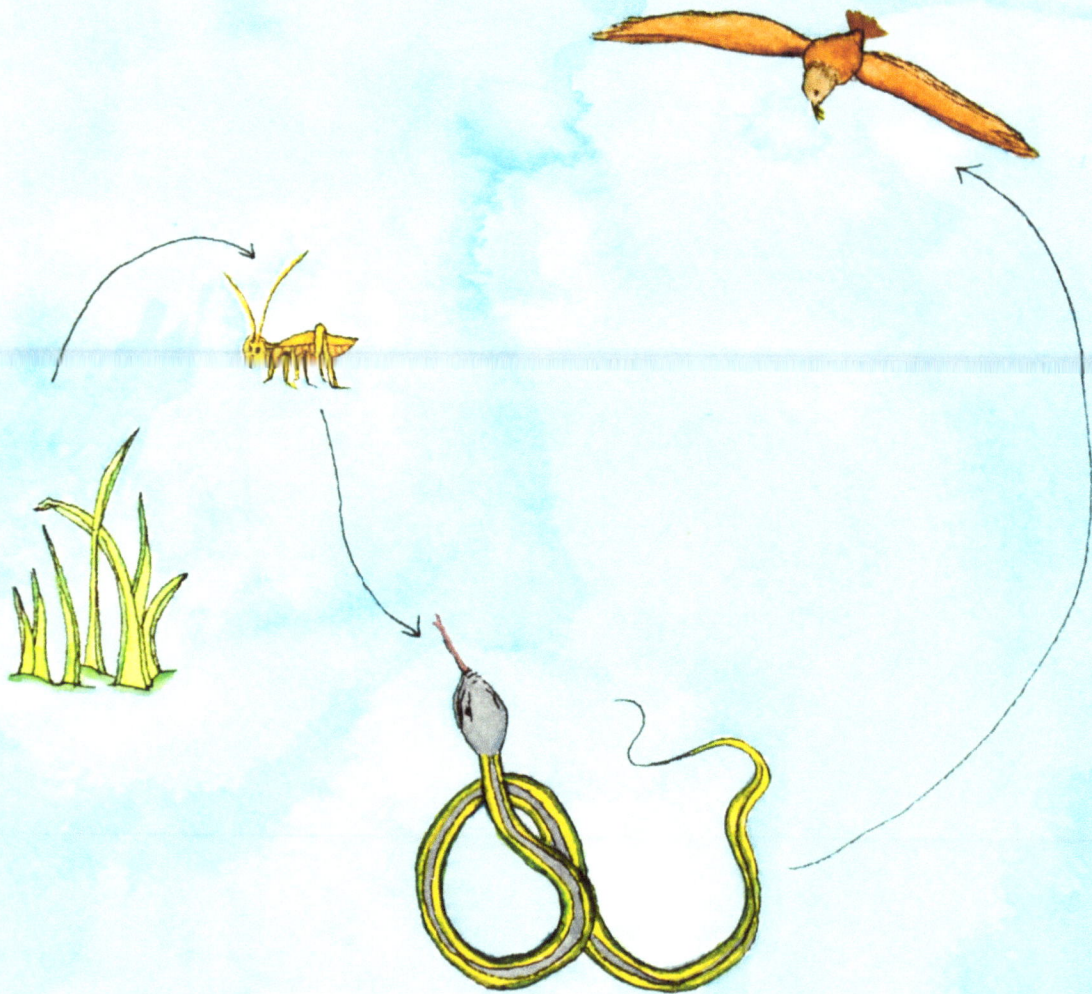

We've all heard about the food chain and how energy flows,

and the cycle continues, that's how everything grows.

The circle of life and the food chain show

how we're all connected, like ribbon for a bow.

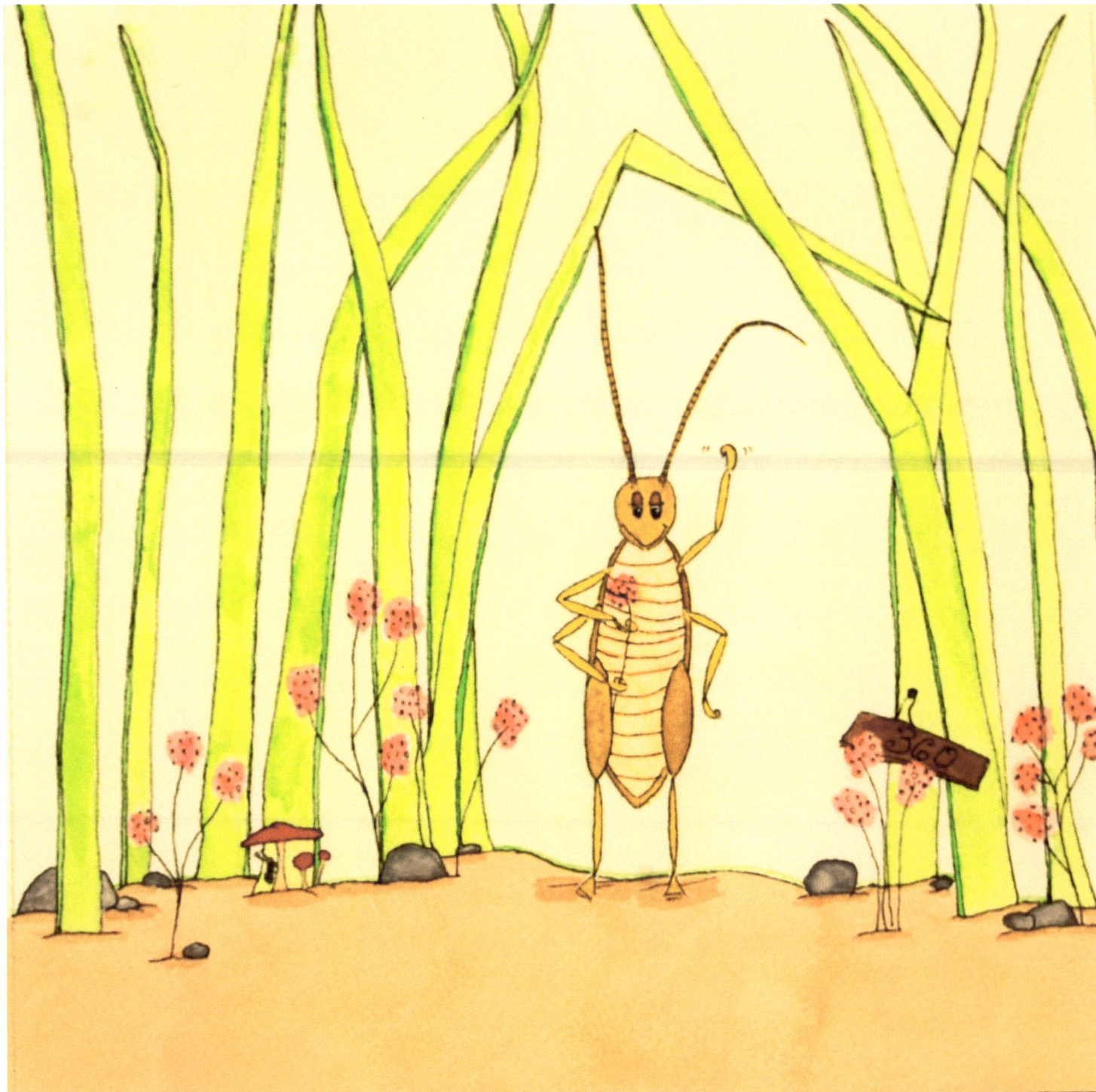

Just one simple decision, no matter how small,

can easily affect grasshopper, mankind and all!

Here is where our story begins,

with a single grasshopper and his two charming friends.

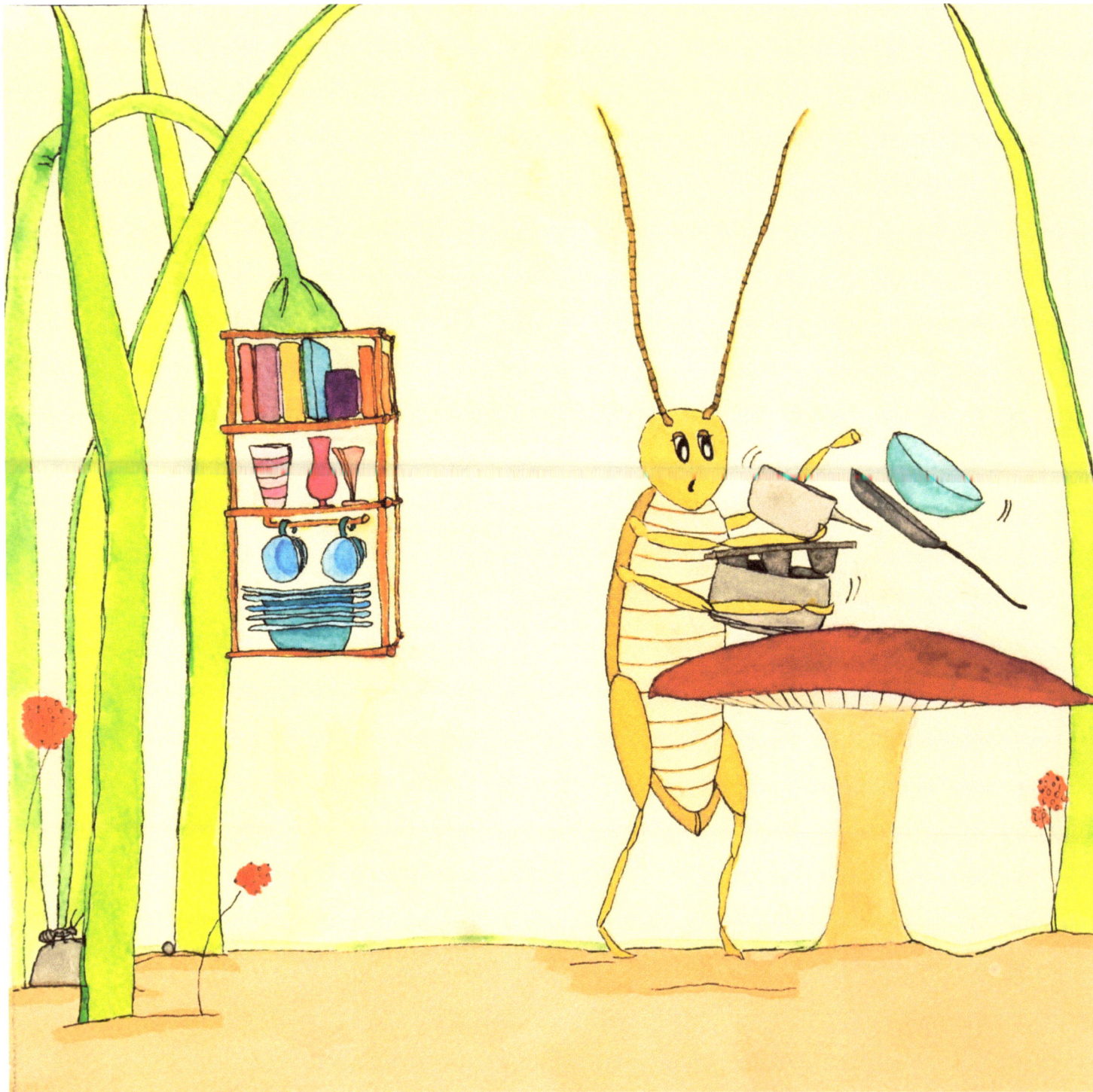

A bit bored with fresh grass, and feeling blue,

he thought long and hard about what he should do.

Then, our friend Grasshopper came up with a plan

to go into his kitchen, and pull out the pans.

He stirred and he mixed and was eager to bake

cupcakes and cookies and chocolate cake!

When the goodies were done, he ate every last one.

He did this for days, until summer was gone.

It wasn't hunger that made grasshopper eat,

but he still craved something delicious and sweet.

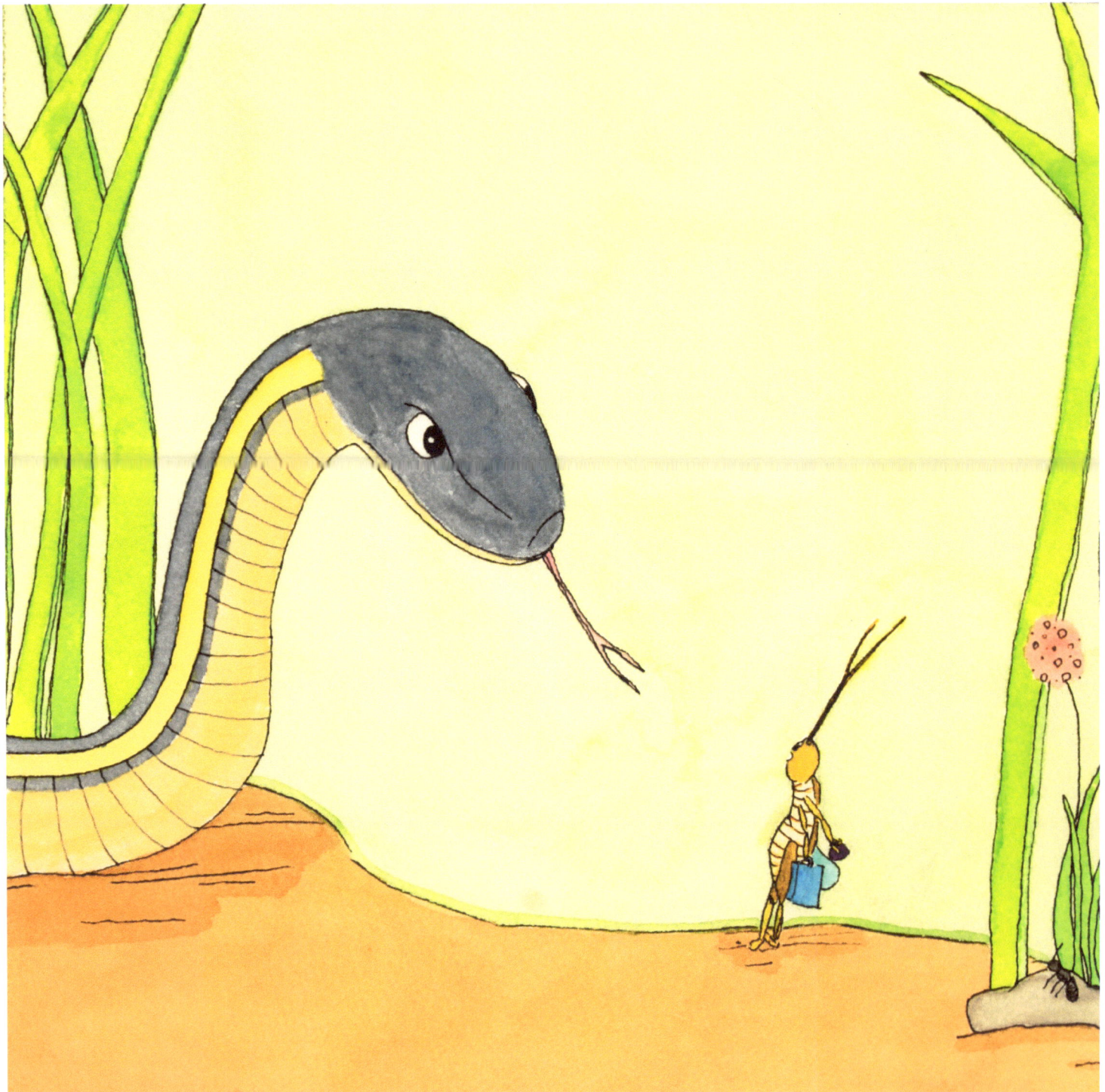

By autumn he felt sleepy and sad when he woke.

Nothing made him smile, not even a joke.

He went for a walk to clear his mind,

but found himself in quite a big bind.

When a snake slithered out from under a bush,

the startled grasshopper fell right on his tush.

"Oh Chubby Grasshopper, what a meal you'll make."

The grasshopper begged, "Please don't! This is a mistake!"

He had to think fast or meet his fate.

If only he had something to use as bait.

As Snake impatiently waited for a reason,

Grasshopper explained, "I've been baking all season."

"If into my den you would just come and see,

I have cupcakes, and cookies and TONS of goodies."

Into Grasshopper's house they did go,

a new found friend where once was a foe.

Grasshopper baked all day and all night.

He and the Snake ate every last bite.

With no grass in sight, but dessert all around,

Snake (like Grasshopper) became very run down.

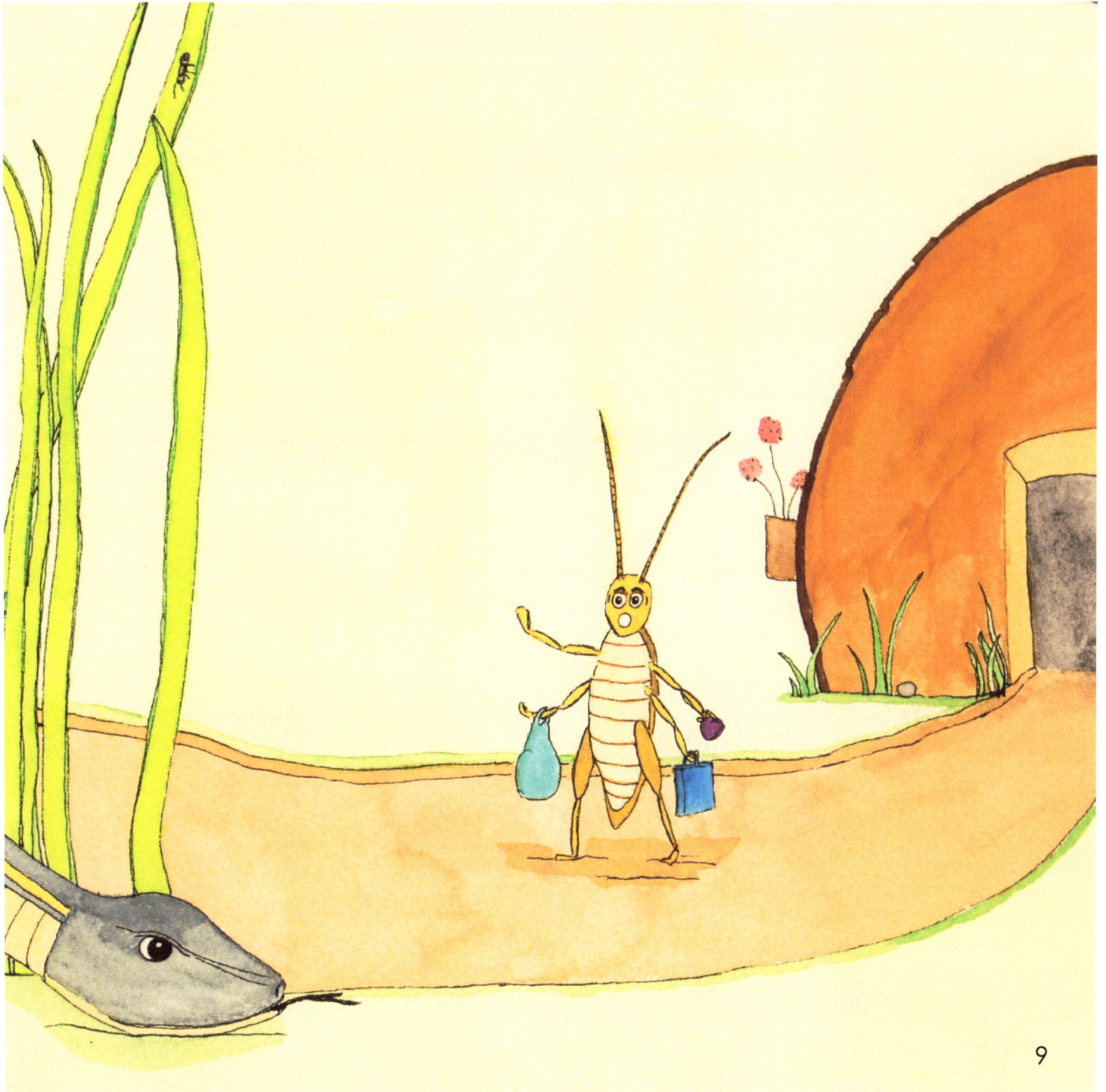

Soon autumn ended and there was a chill in the air.

Snake and Grasshopper just didn't care.

They ate and ate until they could barely move.

The floor where they sat had a permanent groove.

It seemed everyday they were more sluggish and tired.

Baking was the only thing that made them inspired...

to leave the den and buy more sweets;

to make éclairs and brownies and sugary treats.

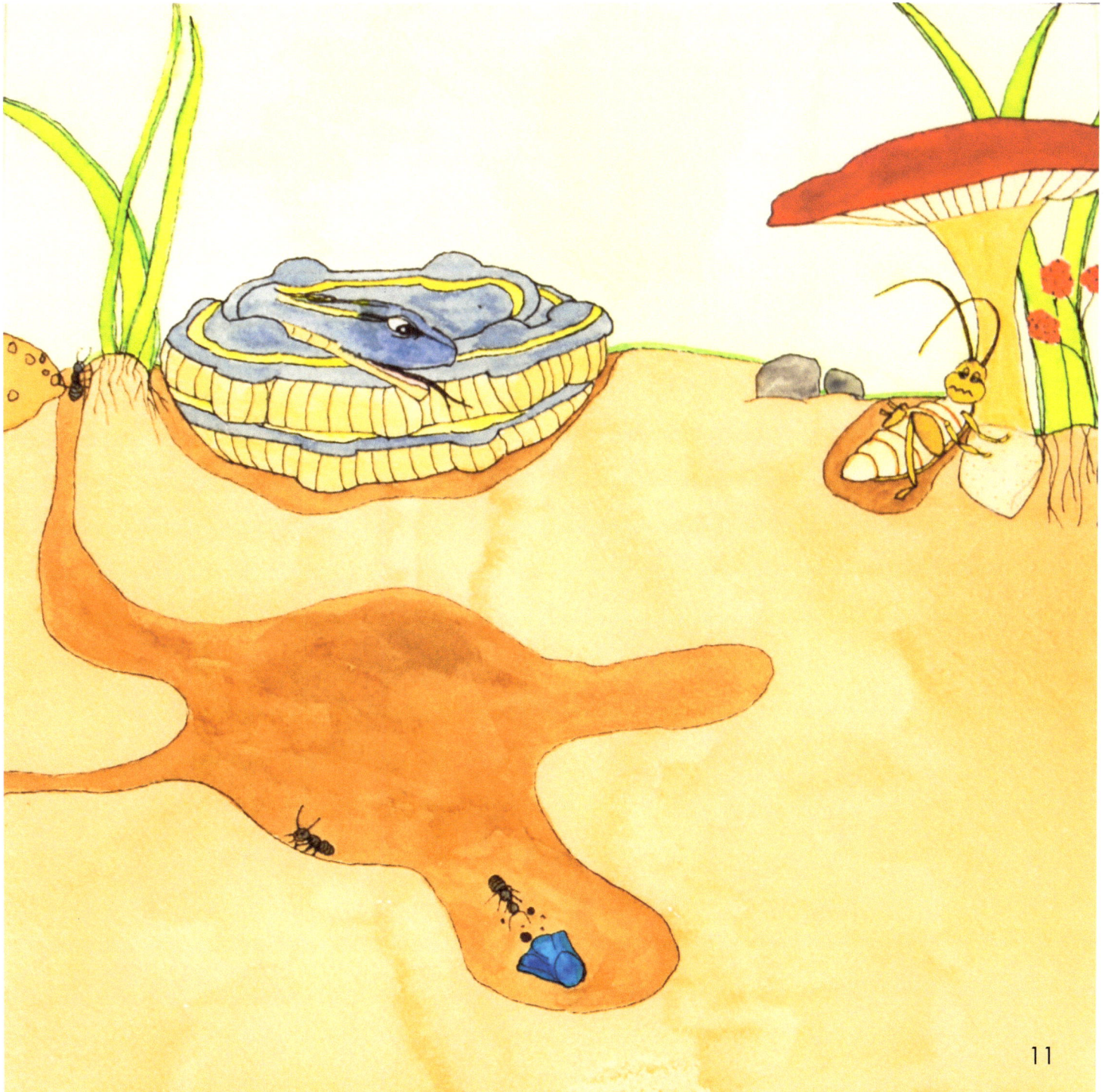

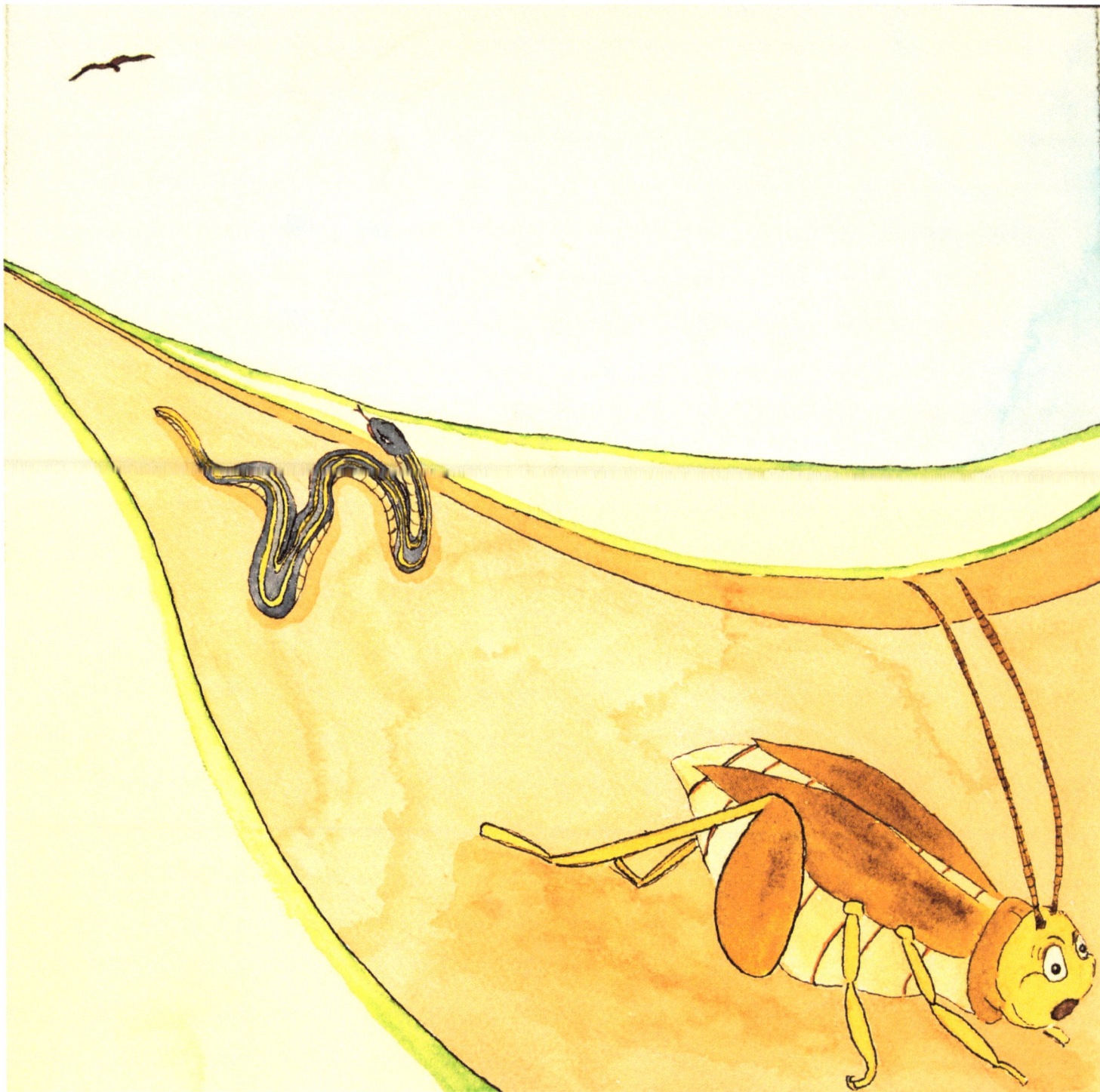

Walking was difficult for our sleepy twosome.

The hike to the store seemed lengthy and gruesome.

As they walked, the sky was cloudy and gray.

So were their minds and their hearts on that day.

They did not have the energy a walk required.

Going a short distance had left them quite tired.

When what should appear with a flutter of wings?

A hawk, of all the horrible things!

Grasshopper and Snake knew it was too late,

to try and run (not that they could) after all that they ate.

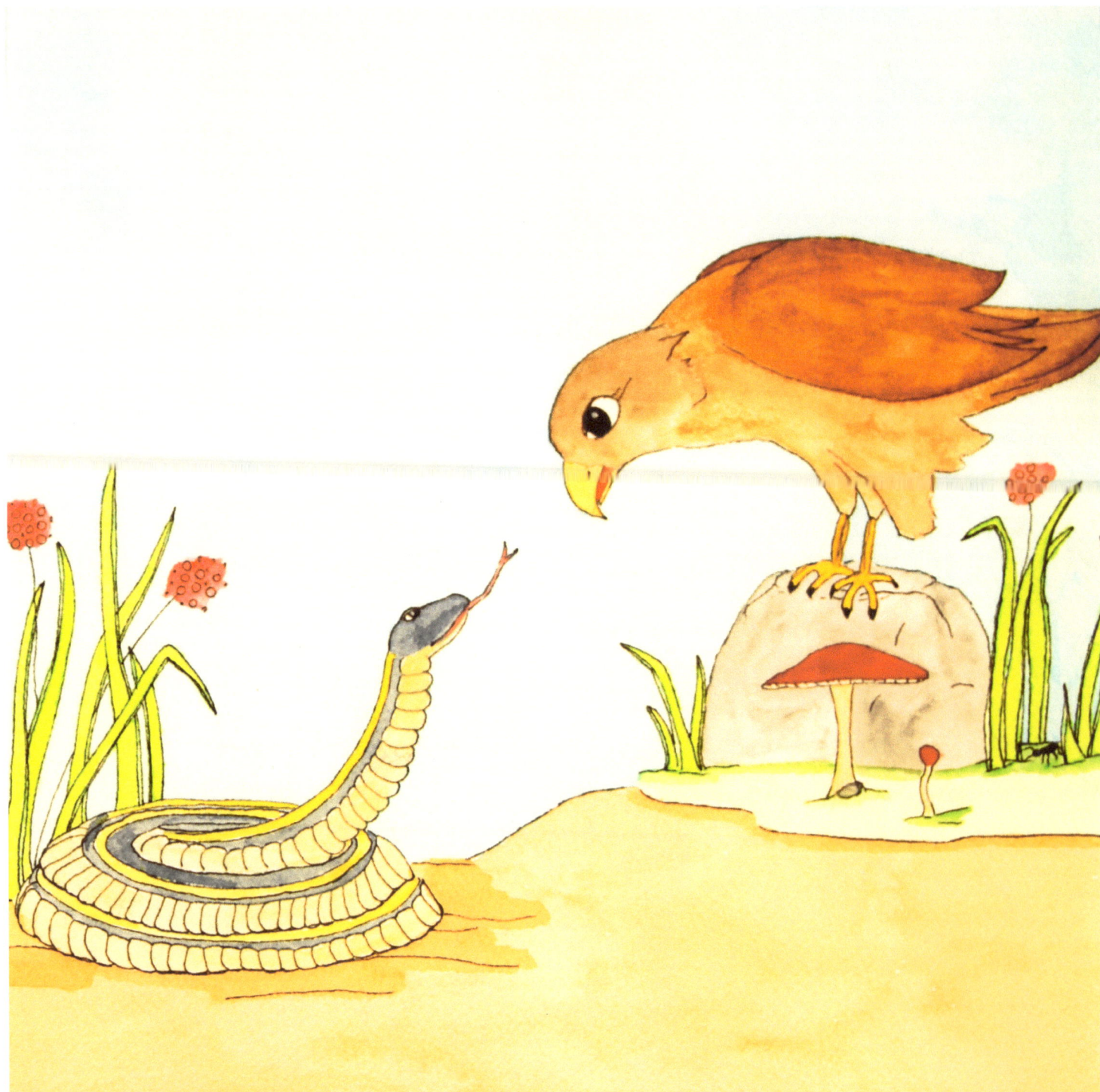

"You are both so plump," said Hawk with a grin.

"Oh well, more food for me. It looks like I win!"

"Please," said Snake, "don't turn us into lunch."

"Don't worry I won't," said Hawk, "it's technically brunch."

"Come back with us now to Grasshopper's den;

we'll make something tastier than **we** would have been."

"I don't know," said Hawk, still unsure.

"I usually only eat food that is pure."

Snake knew he was running out of time.

"Just try one cookie, they're really divine."

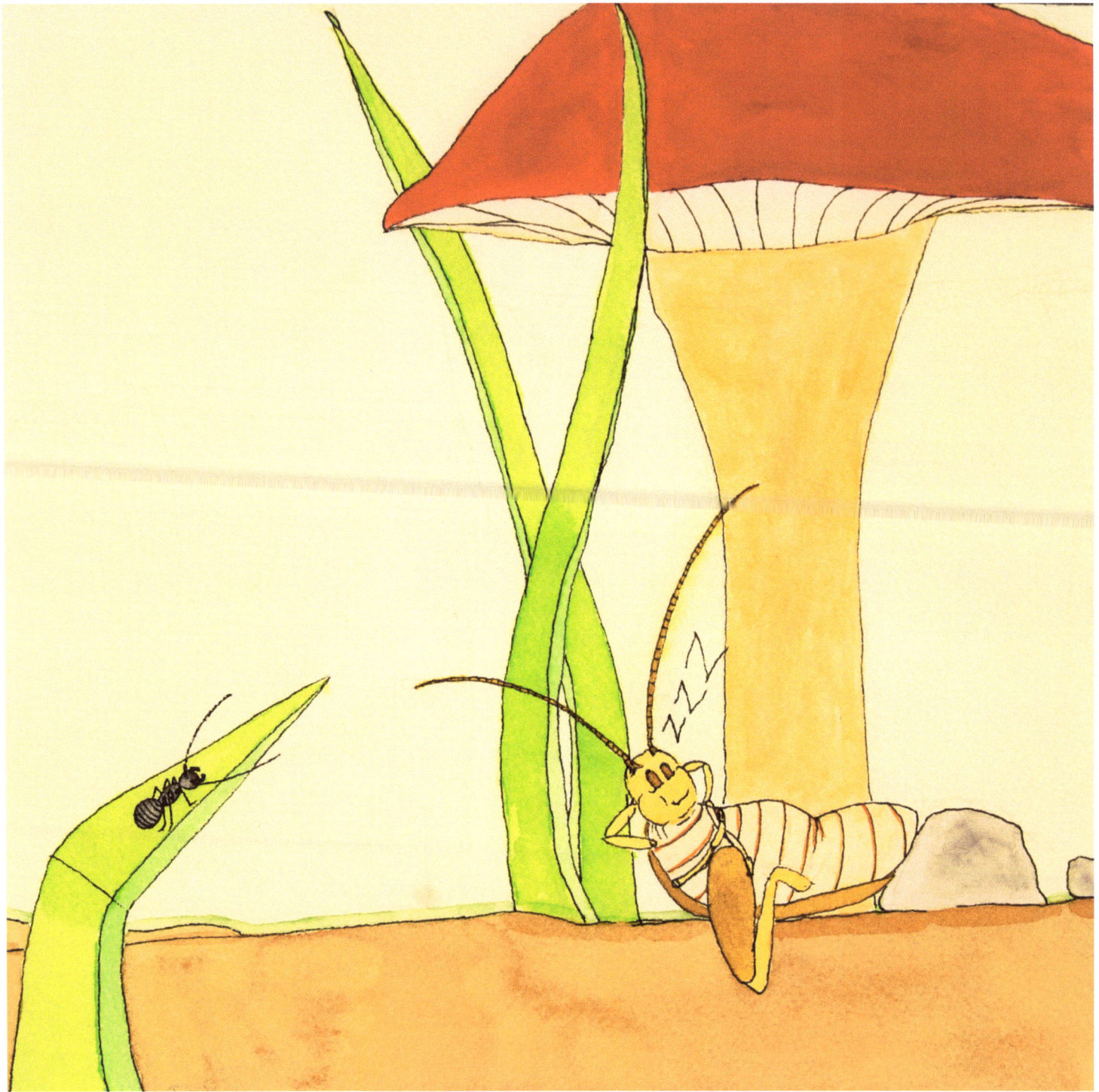

"Fine," said Hawk, in a defeated voice.

Snake sighed with relief, "You made the right choice."

At this point, Grasshopper was quietly snoozing.

Snake did not find this one bit amusing.

"Wake up!" he shouted at his sleeping buddy.

Grasshopper blinked slowly, his mind feeling muddy.

"I must be dreaming, hawks don't eat sweets."

"Neither did we," said Snake, "but now we love treats!"

The three headed home, it was time to start baking.

Hawk never thought about the choice he was making.

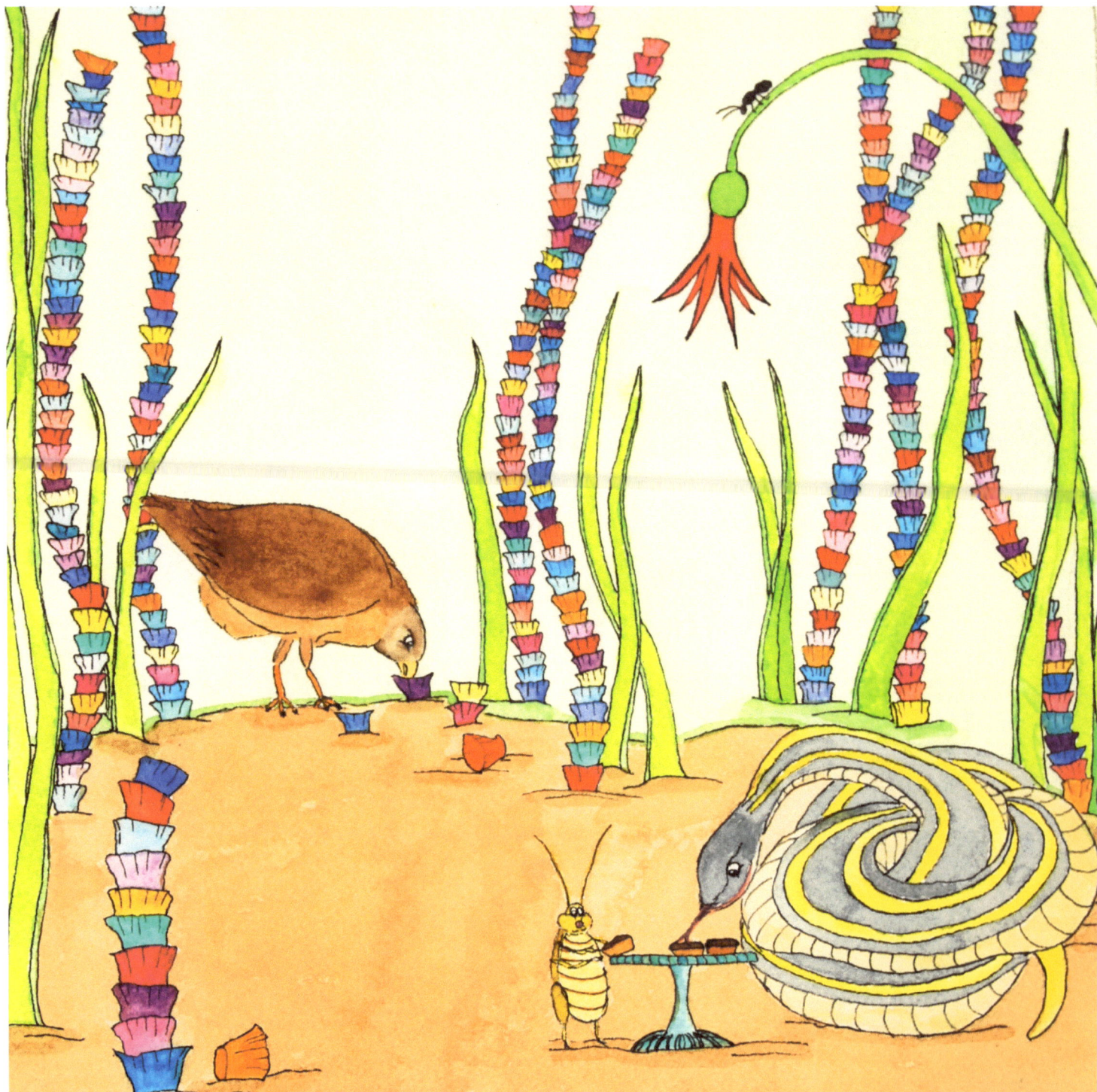

All through the winter, and then it was spring,

the pals baked and ate every last thing.

Until one day, Grasshopper decided he really missed hopping,

he couldn't you know, at least without stopping.

He decided to try and go back to his roots,

eating food for nourishment and energy boosts!

No more muffins or cartons of ice cream,

he returned to the grass so nutritious and green.

He used self-control to decide serving size,

because too much of any food is never wise.

As he became healthy, so too did Snake.

He was able to slither, without needing a break.

Finally, Hawk began to change his ways.

He did miss flying, he hadn't for days.

As his wings fluttered, his heart filled with glee,

he soared through the sky, happy and free.

As the friends made wise choices, they felt more alive.

They felt better and happy and started to thrive.

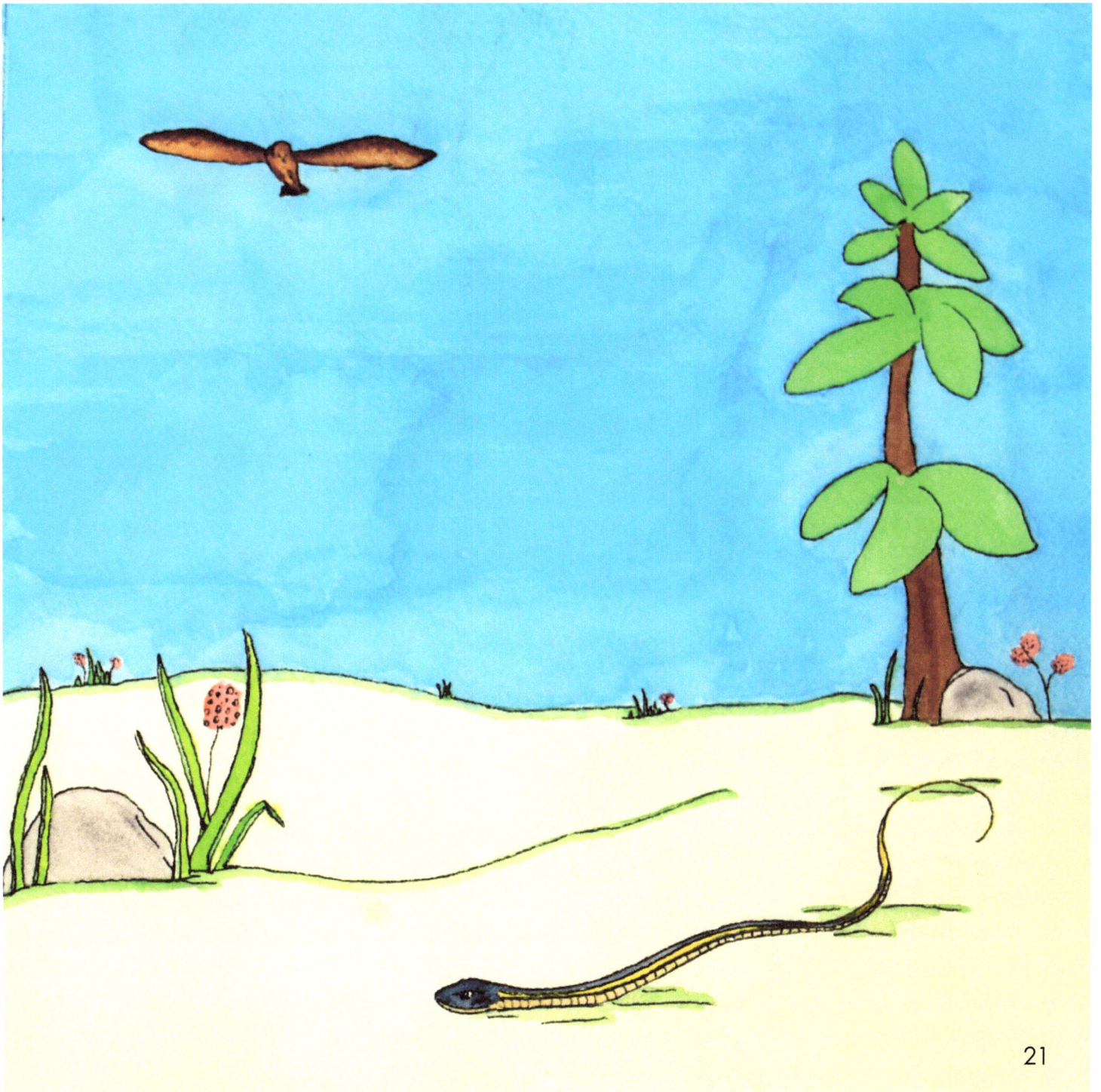

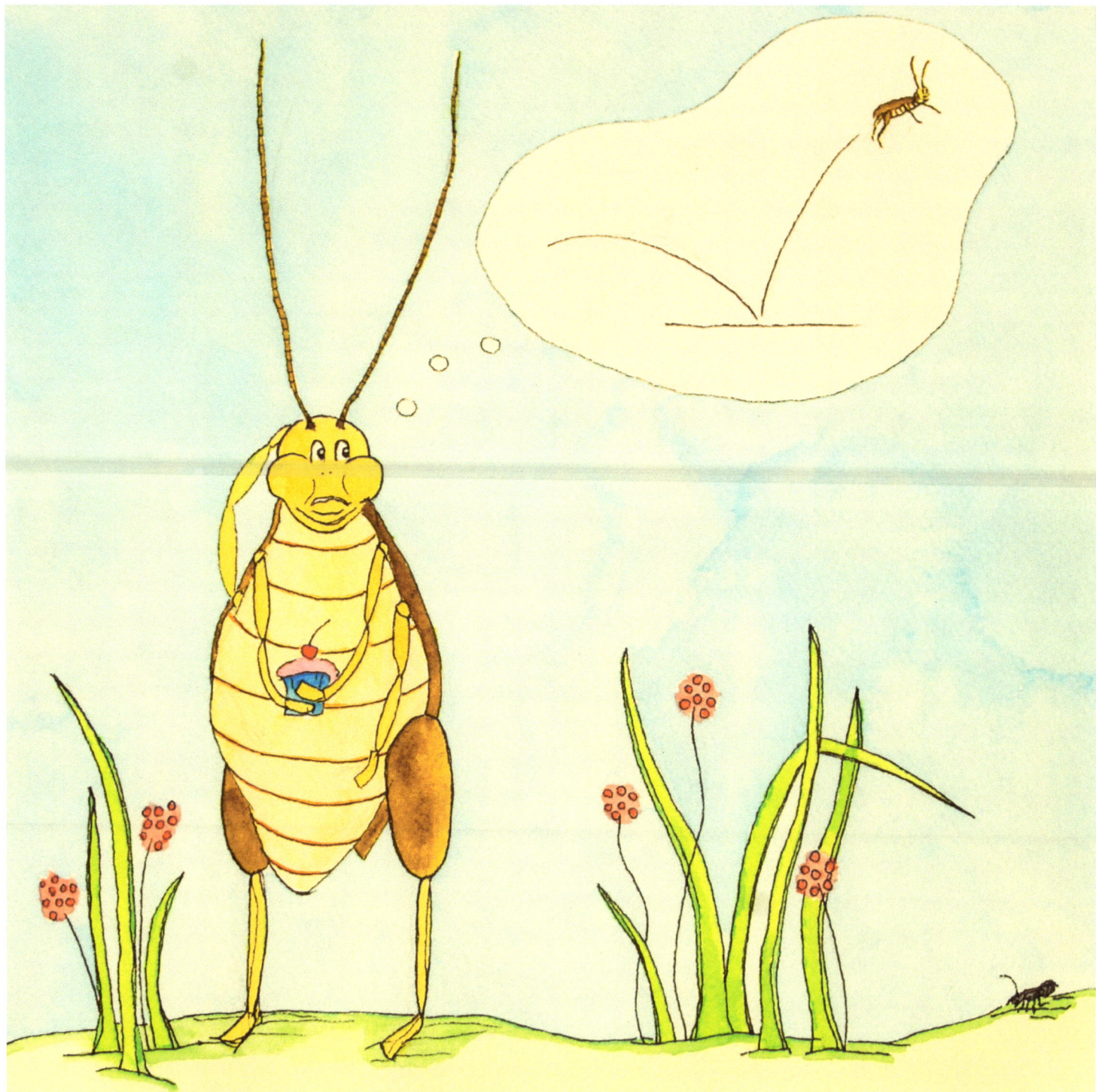

The pals learned that eating the food from the den,

left their bodies struggling, again and again.

If they ate the food, from out in the land,

their bodies felt healthy and perfectly grand!

We learn from each other, these are the facts;

even with something as simple as snacks.

If your friend has a sundae, then you'll want one too.

If my friend has a doughnut, I may buy myself two!

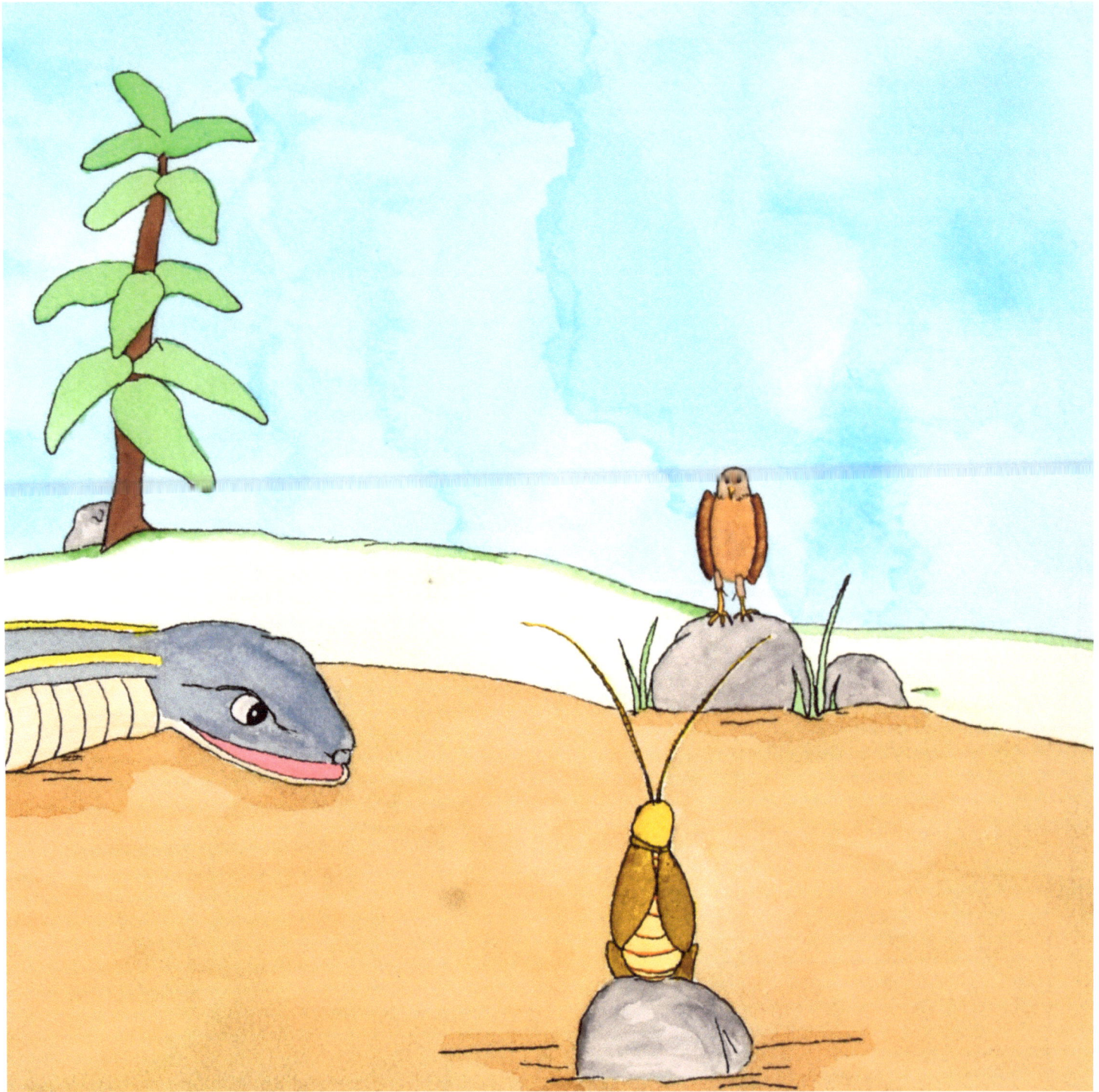

Behaviors are contagious, just like a cold.

"You are what you eat", or so we've been told.

Grasshopper, Snake and Hawk help to show,

how friends and their actions can cause you to grow...

not happy and stronger the way it should be,

but sad and unhealthy...an atrocity!

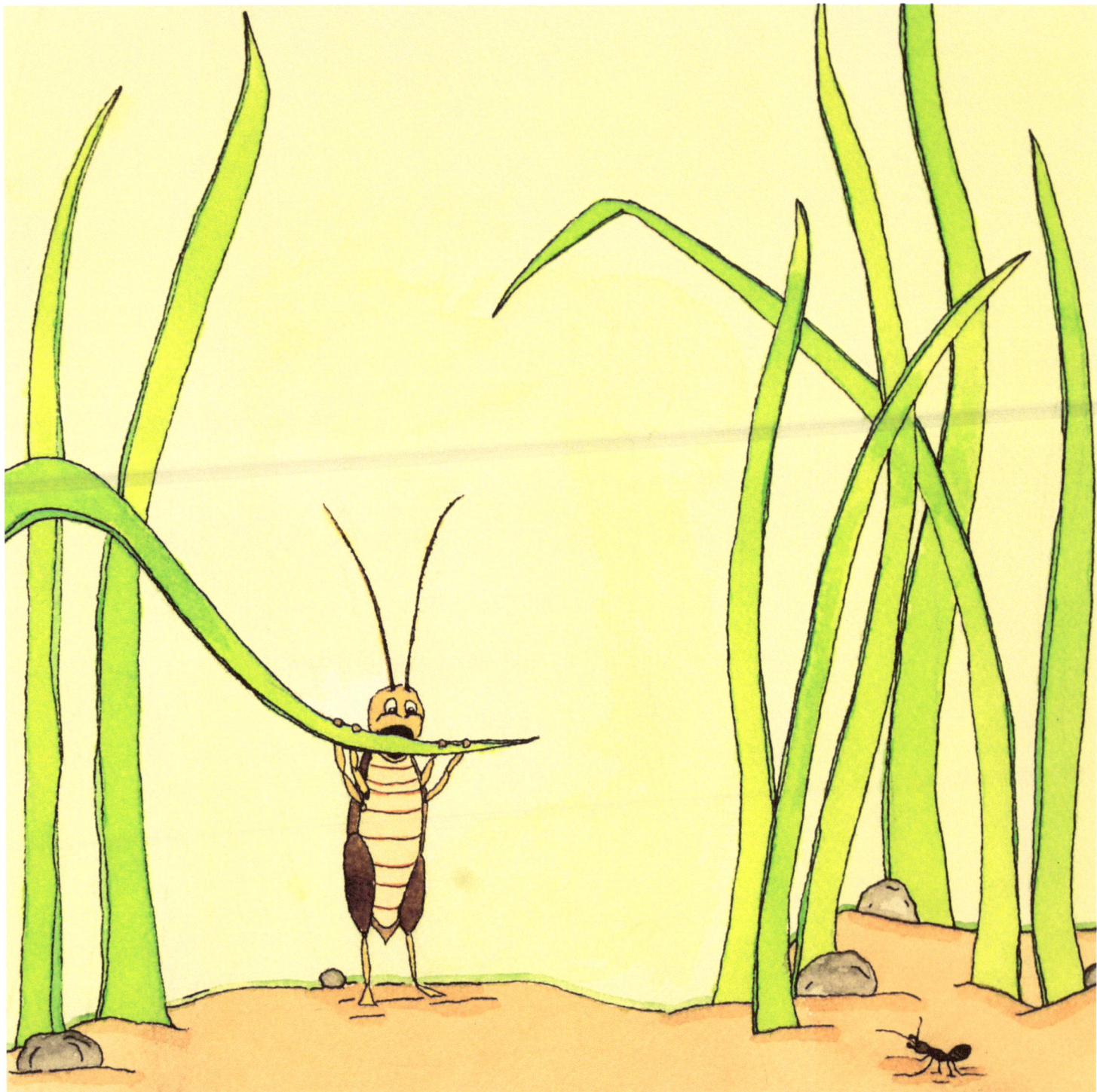

Be sure the next time hunger attacks,

you think before eating and have all the facts.

Your food should be fresh and nutritious to eat.

Share with someone - help the cycle repeat!

Your friends affect you, and you affect them.

We're all connected, grasshopper, snake, hawk and men.

In this beautiful life, there is no "one size fits all",

some are round, some are thin, others short, others tall!

It is never our size that others adore,

but what's on the inside, what's in our core!

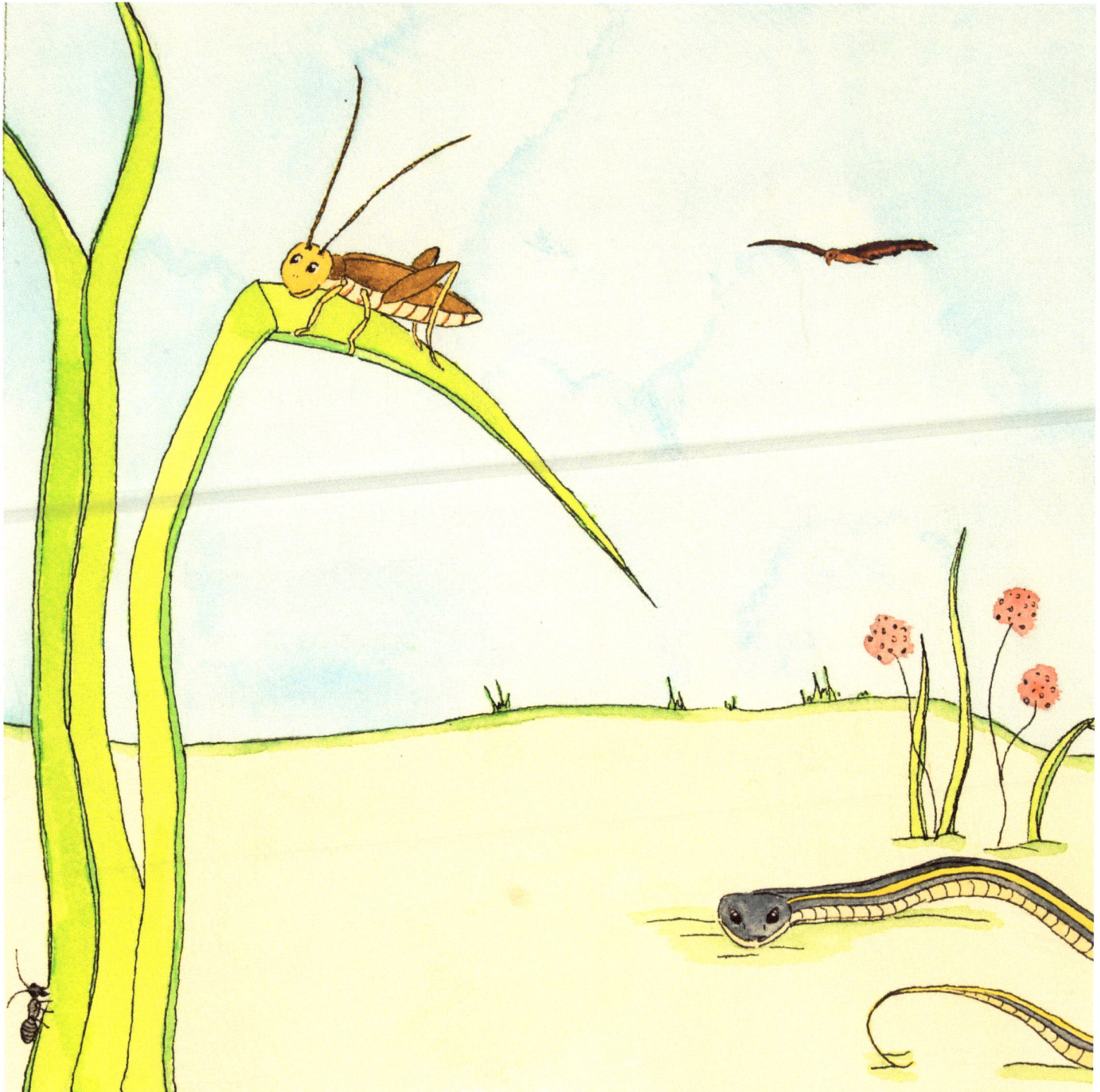

Grasshopper was again hopping and free.

He smiled upon waking, full of energy!

He had come to enjoy eating grass and green food.

It certainly helped improve his blue mood.

Grasshopper exclaimed, "I feel so alive!"

"Now when I eat, I'm fully satisfied."

His two friends smiled with glee!

They too felt renewed and truly happy.

This now brings our story to an end;

the tale of Chubby Grasshopper

and his two charming friends.

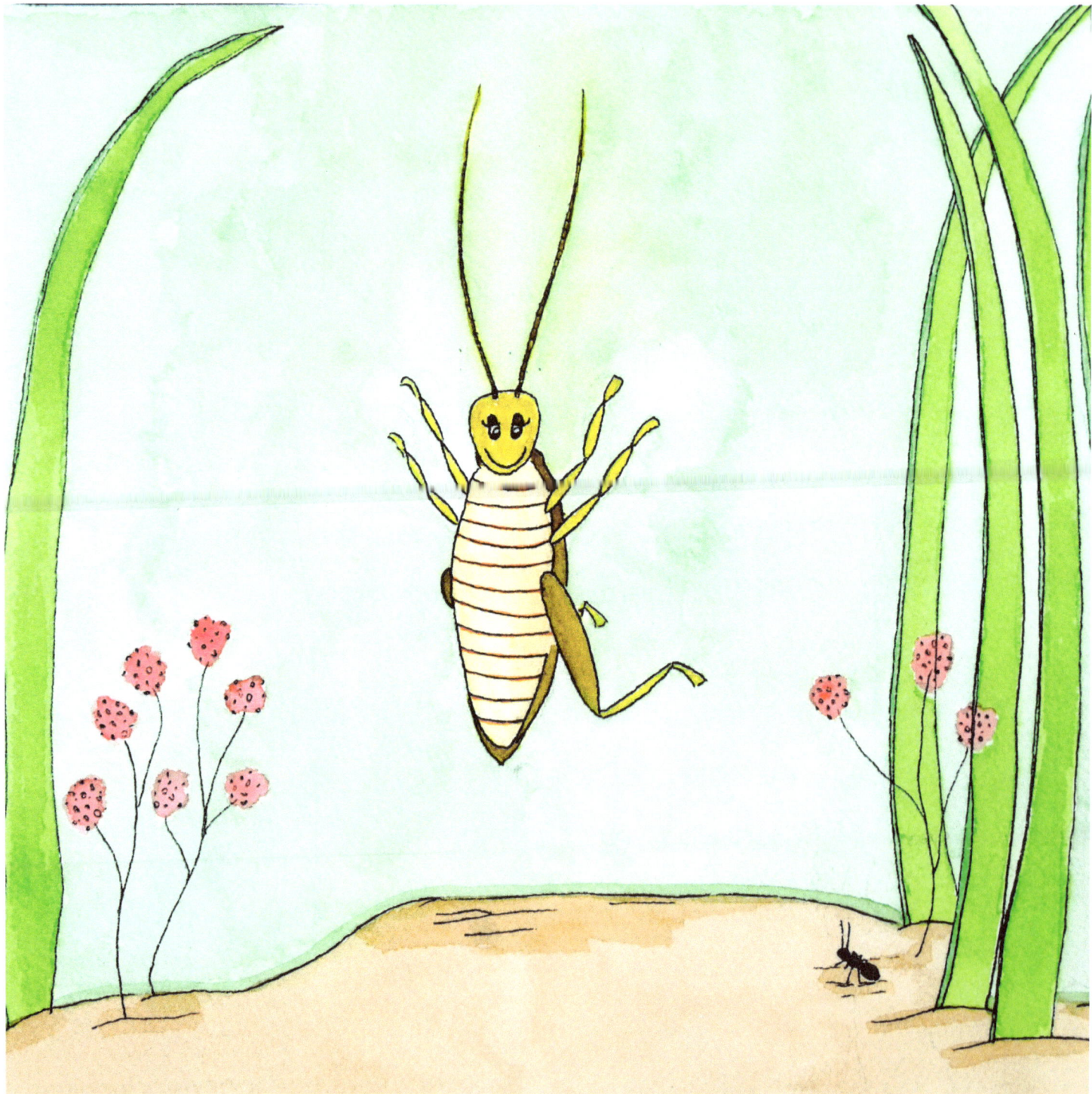

The End

www.ingramcontent.com/pod-product-compliance
Lightning Source LLC
Chambersburg PA
CBHW060834270326
41933CB00002B/86